The Truth about Essential Oils

How to Reap the Benefits of Essential Oil Treatments

By: Patricia Young

Publishers Notes

Disclaimer

Digital Edition

WHAT YOU WILL LEARN IN THIS BOOK

How This Book Will Help You and Why

Many persons have heard the word aromatherapy buy really do not know what the process entails. This book not only provides a brief history of what aromatherapy is and how it originated but it also goes into greater detail. It also focuses on essential oils and shows the link between the use of these oils and aromatherapy.

As in days of old, the book also outlines some of the main things that persons use essential oils for such as to help with certain ailments, to enhance wellbeing and for cosmetic purposes.

Dive Right into the Book! Or Learn a Bit More About the Author

TABLE OF CONTENTS

CHAPTER 1- AN OVERVIEW OF AROMATHERAPY

Whilst the term "Aromatherapy" and its modern day practice comes from the French word "Aromatherapie" coined in 1928 by Professor Rene-Maurice Gattefosse the use of the healing properties of plants dates back many thousands of years. Ancient peoples such as the Australian Aborigines and African Bushmen have long understood plant properties and utilized them in their day to day living.

Even the Old Testament refers to aromatherapy in a holy anointing oil recipe containing myrrh, cinnamon, cassia and calamus that was given to Moses.

Recorded use of plant oils trace the origins of aromatherapy back to civilizations such as the Egyptians, Babylonians, Chinese and Indians in various social, medicinal, religious and personal practices.

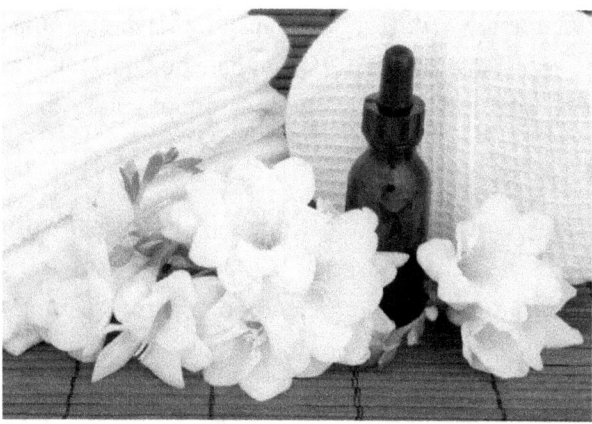

It is the Egyptians who are generally held to have been the first civilization who fully exploited the physical and spiritual properties of aromatic oils between 4000 to 6000 years ago: initially for preserving bodies during the process of mummification and aiding their journey to the after world and later as treatment for the living.

Ancient Egyptians used substances, scents and oils of specific plants in many of their religious ceremonies and rituals including embalming, purifying, fumigating, cleansing, healing and beautifying. Myrrh was burned at dawn as an offering to the moon and frankincense was offered to the sun.

They were also well versed in other uses of aromatherapy and used it into their cooking; specific herbs helped build the immune system, protected against infection and helped the digestive process.

Cleopatra is credited with intimate knowledge of the use of aromatherapy for the seduction of men through the use of essential oils in cosmetic practices.

Ayurveda, a traditional Indian medicine has been practiced for about 3000 years. Early Ayurvedic writings show ancient knowledge of aromatherapy with detailed recordings of the use of sandalwood, jasmine, spikenard and rose essential oils and incorporating essential oils into their healing potions.

The herbal book written by Shen Nung's is the oldest existing medical book in China, it is dated around 2700 B.C. is and it is filled with information on more than three hundred plants. The Ancient Chinese used sweet-smelling herbs and burned incense and aromatic woods as a sign of respect to their God.

Clay tablets dating back to 1800 B.C. recording the use of cedar wood have been discovered from the Babylonian civilization.

Both the medicinal and cosmetic properties of aromatic oils were initially passed on to the Greeks from the Egyptians. Hippocrates the "Father of Modern Medicine" wrote widely on the effects of some 300 plants including cumin, marjoram, peppermint, saffron and thyme. Hippocrates extensive knowledge of plants and their essences was Ayurvedic in origin and was gained through the Greek soldiers encounters with Ayurvedic medicine on the Indian sub-continent during their campaigns with Alexander the Great. Hippocrates and his students believed Ayurveda was harmonious with their own medicinal practices.

Hippocrates wrote "a perfumed bath and a scented massage everyday is the way to good health". He also wrote what many believe to be the most important principle in modern medicine "Above all, the purpose of a doctor is to awaken the natural healing energies within the body"

Other Greeks who contributed to the knowledge of the properties in essential oils used in aromatherapy included Theophrastus, Herodotus and Democretus.

Galen was another Greek whose immense knowledge of plants and their medicines had a lasting impact on how we classify information today. He began as a surgeon at a school for gladiators and during Galen's term as physician it is claimed that no gladiator died of his wounds. His reputation spread far and wide and he was eventually promoted to the position of personal physician to the Roman Emperor, Marcus Aurelius. He wrote extensively on the theory of plant medicine and divided plants into various medicinal categories that are still known as "Galenic" today.

The Roman Empire saw the widespread use of essential oils for massage, in scented baths, bedding, and clothing and to scent their hair. Although the fall of the Roman empire caused the use of essential oils to die out in Europe the practice flourished elsewhere such as in Arabia where in about

1000 A.D. the physician Ali-Ibn Sana, known as Avicenna the Arab, is credited with being the first to distil rose essence. He wrote on over 800 medicinal plants and included many aromatics including rose, lavender and chamomile.

Knights returning from the Crusades in the Middle East carried perfumes and passed on the knowledge they had acquired on herbal medicines and distillation throughout Western Europe.

Although knowledge of essential oils died out in Europe the antiseptic and anti-bacterial properties of plants was still recognized as evidenced in the burning of herbal woods such as pine and Frankincense to ward off evil spirits and for fumigation. During the Bubonic Plague of the 14th Century it was noted that less people died of the plague in the areas where this was done.

By the 17th century, herbalism had a massive revival during which a number of books on herbs, called herbals, were written, including the works of John Gerard and Nicholas Culpepper, where therapeutic properties of plants were recorded. These documents lay the foundations for modern day aromatherapy.

The French pharmacist Professor Rene-Maurice Gattefosse is recognized as defining "Aromatherapie" as a result of accidentally plunged his burnt hand into lavender oil and found that his hand healed quickly without blistering or scaring. His book "Aromatherapie" was published in 1928 in which he details cases of essential oils and their healing capabilities.

This work was continued and extended by Dr Jean Valnet who treated a number of conditions such as tuberculosis, diabetes and other serious conditions with essential oils and claimed a number of success stories. He also used essential oils as antiseptics to treat soldiers in World War II.

An Austrian biochemist Marguerite Maury developed the method of applying essential oils through aromatherapy massage over the course of the 1900's and pioneered work on the application of aromatherapy to health care and beauty therapy, studying the way in which essential oils work both physically and emotionally.

The pioneering works of aromatherapy have all contributed to the fantastic body of knowledge that exists today and has helped make aromatherapy one of the fastest growing complementary therapies of our modern age.

It is extensively used at hospitals, in clinics and in homes for a number of applications like helping to rehabilitate cardiac patients, alleviate the pain cancer patients experience from chemotherapy and to ease women's labor pains.

Just as Feng Shui did, aromatherapy is slowly making its way into mainstream business. For example, in Japan engineers are placing aromatic systems into recently constructed buildings. So the aroma of rosemary and lavender is pumped into the waiting area for customers to soothe the customers, while the scents from lemon As well as eucalyptus is utilized in the banks to keep the staff attentive.

Aromatherapy & Essential Oils

Each essential oil has a distinctive make-up resulting in a range of qualities. The three hundred or so essences have anti-bacterial, antiseptic, anti-viral, uplifting, calming, and diuretic, anti spasmodic; cell rejuvenating properties to name a few and any single essential oil can host a range of those qualities.

Pure undulated essential oils contain tiny molecules that are easily absorbed through the skin, making them ideal for aromatherapy treatments. Aromatherapy works on both the physical level through the known medicinal and scientific properties and on the psychological level through the emotional response triggered by the actual scents of each essential oil. Aromatherapy treatments administer essential oils externally through the direct contact with the skin by massage and bathing and also through the olfactory senses by means of diffusers or inhalation.

By having the ability to calm, uplift, ease tension and reduce anxiety, amongst others, essential oils are ideally suited to helping us with our modern day stress filled lifestyles by providing us with a holistic approach to treating mind, body and spirit.

CHAPTER 2- WHAT ARE THE BENEFITS OF ESSENTIAL OILS?

The Prime Benefits of Using Essential Oils

A major physical benefit to essential oils is they help to fight foreign elements known for causing the body unwanted harm. Most of these oils have anti-bacteria properties to them. When you bathe in these oils, the microbes in the oils can go to work attacking bacteria which, in turn, means the oils can help reduce problems with infections. While not a cure-all to every problem someone might have, even a small amount of infection prevention is going to be a major positive.

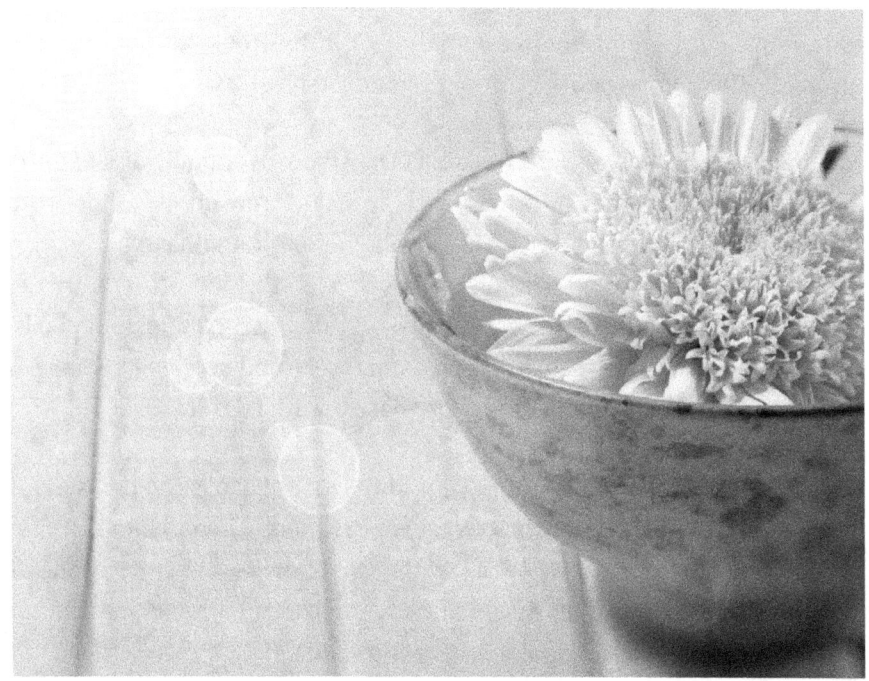

Essentially oils also have an anti-fungal aspect to them. Fungi not exactly anyone's friend when it causes problems for the body. A natural element capable of reducing the presence of fungi on the skin is most assuredly going to be appreciated by those stressing out over fungus in the toenails and elsewhere.

Antioxidants are extremely helpful as a means of boosting one's health to optimal levels. Free radicals are always seeking to attack the cells of the human body, which is why a diet rich in antioxidants is so strongly recommended. The one thing to be aware of when it comes to antioxidants is they do not solely have to be acquired through dietary means. Yes, antioxidants can be absorbed through the skin via essential oils. In fact, essential oils are a tremendous source of these powerful antioxidants.

It is worth mentioning that essential oils can also help to enhance cell strength. The human body is comprised of millions of cells.

Steam, of course, travels into the air. While steam eventually dissipates in the air, any materials it brings with it might remain. In short, the molecules of the essential oils can remain in the air and have a purifying effect on it. Human beings, of course, inhale the air present in the environment in which they dwell. Thanks to the presence of essential oils, the quality of the air can improve immensely and this might have a number of beneficial health effects on those breathing the air.

The calming effect of the natural scent of the essential oils can be used for relaxation and stress reduction. Yes, there are mental health benefits that can be gained from slowly inhaling the scent of these oils. No one is suggesting, however that essential oils are the preferable method of treating serious anxiety conditions. For those dealing with more than a bit of stress, essential oils can offer a contribution to a much needed calming effect.

The delivery method of the essential oils should never be dismissed when examining all the benefits associated with the oils. Essential oils can penetrate the pores of the skin quite easily.

CHAPTER 3- HOW TO USE, ACQUIRE AND STORE ESSENTIAL OILS

Essential oils have been around for centuries. They smell good and provide a number of therapeutic benefits. Surprisingly, they are not oils but the liquid extract of plants. While there are a few ways to produce essential oils, the most common method is steam distillation. In this method, hot steam is used extract the oil from the plant. The steam is then cooled and the essential oil is separated from the water. The other common methods are cold pressing and solvent extraction. Cold pressing is pressing the oil out of the plant. Solvent extraction is using a solvent to extract the oil from the plant. This is often used when a plant has a low yield of essential oil.

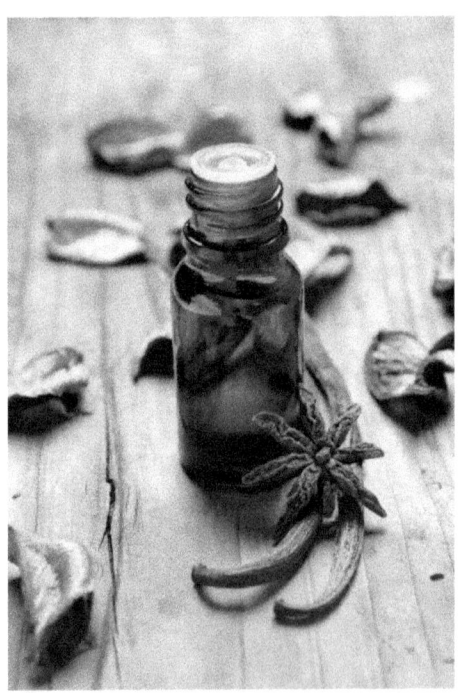

Essential oils are highly concentrated. Each oil carries many of the properties of the plant from which it was extracted, including scent and medicinal properties. A large number of plants are required to extract a small amount of oil. The amount varies depending on the plant. For example, it takes a whopping 4,000 pounds of Bulgarian roses to produce one pound of oil. On the other hand, it takes 100 pounds of lavender to produce a pound of oil. Thus, prices can range from $700 for two fluid ounces of Bulgarian Rose essential oil to $16 for two fluid ounces of lavender essential oil.

Essential oils have an extremely long shelf life, ranging from two to ten years. And because a little goes a long way, a small bottle would likely suffice for a long time. Essential oils are used frequently in aromatherapy. They are also often used in soaps and creams, waxes, butters and alcohols. Because they are concentrated, most essential oils should be diluted prior to applying to the skin. If essential oils are used directly on the skin, they can cause burning, photosensitivity or skin irritation. Essential oils also need to be kept away from eyes and out of the reach of young children and pets. Pregnant women also need to be careful when handling essential oils.

Essential oils must always be bought from a supplier that is not only well known but reputable as well. This supplier must have in stock the best quality therapeutic oils. There are lower grade essential oils that can be purchased but they will not have the same therapeutic effect in the long run.

It is important to keep essential oils pure by making sure they are never exposed to contaminants, or adulterated by unethical distillers. Many oils are produced by distillers for the flavor and fragrance industries, so they are not concerned with keeping the essential oils pure the way that is preferred for aromatherapy use. That is also why it is better to buy aromatherapy-grade essential oil from a trusted, reputable source, rather than a random reseller who probably does not have enough experience to even know the difference.

Low-grade oils have little, if any, therapeutic benefits, so for aromatherapy to work you must find a trusted, educated source and then make sure to keep your essential oils pure by storing them properly in amber colored glass away from continuous exposure to heat and UV light.

Not all plants produce an aromatic essence called essential oil. This essence is often therapeutic, but the essential oil is considered to be a part of the plants immune system, and as a defense some plants produce essential oils with toxic compounds. So just because something is an essential oil does not automatically mean it is used in traditional aromatherapy. Even some oils that are topically therapeutic should never be ingested, like eucalyptus or patchouli. It is important to understand the ways that different oils are used to know whether they should only be used topically in dilution, and if there are any contraindications with other health concerns.

CHAPTER 4- WHAT IS THE BEST WAY TO BLEND ESSENTIAL OILS?

Nothing soothes the soul and senses more like creating the perfect blend using your own mix of essential oils. In fact essential oils have a number of great benefits that can bring all kinds of enjoyment into your surroundings, however, many can be toxic or cause allergic reactions so caution must be taken. Gathering essential oils and creating a specific blend can be used for aromatherapy and also for medicinal purposes as well. In order to know what types of oils you are going to blend you will first have to decide what you will actually be blending these oils for. You may be looking for oils to give you an energy boost of you may be looking for something that soothes the spirit, perhaps even send good luck your way. More importantly, you will need to decide if you are using essential oils internally or externally.

Organic essential oils are grouped together by their aromas and oils that are from the same "families" typically yield the best smells and results. Some of the categories for aromatherapy include Earthy, Floral, Woodsy, Minty, Herbaceous, Medicinal, Oriental, Spicy, and Citrus. Essential oils can also be blended together with several other groups to add a different effect. For example, you can blend Spicy and Oriental family or mix together a Floral and Minty family to create different scents adding a touch of citrus to give you a more varied combination of effects. When you select the specific essential oils to your liking then you can go into the testing phase to see which blends make the perfect combination based on your own uses for them.

Some of the most relaxing blends are composed of lavender and chamomile. Other essential oil blends may generate an uplifting feeling and this is best left in the hands of lemon and bergamot. There are many categories that essentials oil can be included in such as:

- Emotional well being
- Skincare, beauty and hygiene
- Physical well-being
- Seasonal
- Household purification and freshening

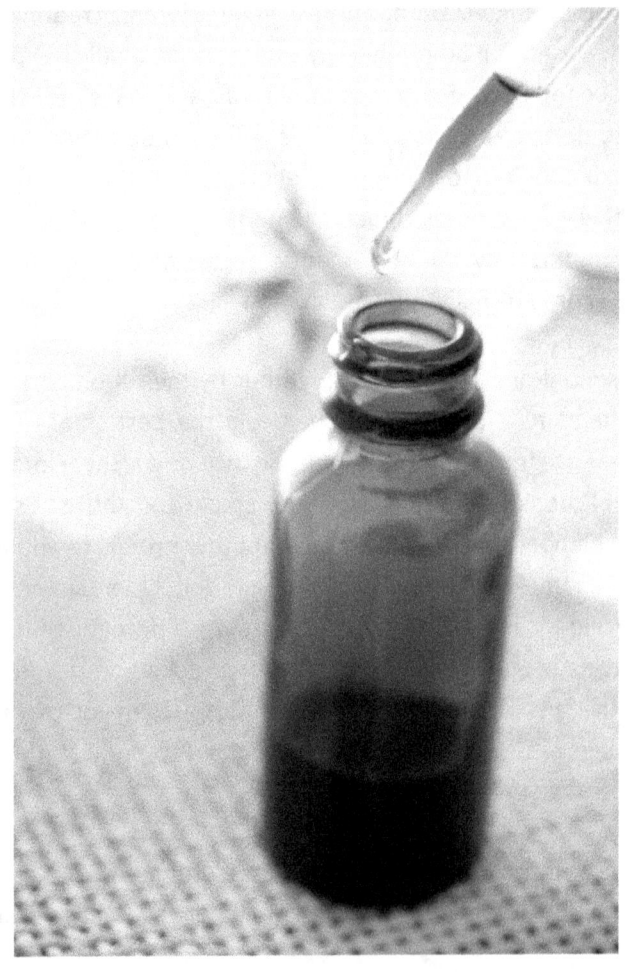

The whole idea of blending essential oils is considered a science and art form all mixed into one bottle so to speak. For example, the chemistry composition of certain essential oils will decide all of its properties, including how violable and viscous it will be. These types of properties should be considered ahead of time before you start blending essential oils.

Many oils start off very thin in their viscosity, meaning they are water-like in their consistency. Others like balsams, resins and absolutes can be nearly solid when they are at room temperature and may be harder to work and blend with. The essential oil scent can also be affected by the order in which the oils are placed. For blending essential oils, it is best to use utensils that are non-metallic and try to stay away from materials such as plastic if you can help it. One of the best materials to use for blending essential oils is glass. These can be glass droppers or glass rods.

Before you start blending it is important to take note that 10 drops of essential oil is recommended for blending. You should become aware of particular blends that you are not quite fond of and ones that are just what you are looking for. Once you have gathered and mixed your blend, you can let it sit aside for 24 to 48 hours max. This period is known as a resting phase and it allows the essential oils to mix well together making your blend better. Some of the most relaxing blends are composed of mixtures that include lavender and chamomile. Other oils may generate uplifting qualities in their mixtures.

The very last step with blending your essential oils would be to test your blend. In this test you will see if you like the aroma. If you find the scent pleasant you can add carrier oils such as Jojoba, Grape-seed, Avocado, or Sweet Almond to dilute them. For good measure and further dilution, you can add five more drops of any chosen carrier oil to your blend. If you do in fact find this scent to be satisfactory you can make another blend with larger amounts this time in the next batch.

Some important things to also note is that, when you blend your essential oils you should store them in the proper environment so that they can function like they are supposed to. This means that all bottles should be sealed tightly and stored in a cool location out of direct sunlight. Some essential oils can be poisonous and should be kept away from children and pets as well. They should also not be placed anywhere near sparks or flames as some of them are quite flammable. Oils like peppermint and fir will catch fire quite quickly as an example. Air spaces should be left within the bottles as well so that the oil is able to "breathe." If you decide to use carrier oil you should fill the container about half-way, then place your essential oil inside. After this, add the rest of the carrier oil turning it over several times to mix.

You also may wonder what would happen if you accidently mixed the wrong oils. This all depends on what you are blending. There is always room for improvements which is why it is recommended to do the smaller blends first.

An example of a typical essential oil blend for helping out individuals with arthritis would include:

- A Carrier Oil
- Roman Chamomile
- Helichrysum

This blend for arthritis should be mixed together well and placed in an air-tight container that is dark colored. There are also several carrier oils that have anti-inflammatory properties that you can add to the blend.

Pomegranate Seed, Hemp Seed, and Jojoba Oils are great for this particular effect, although other carries may not be.

CHAPTER 5- BEST ESSENTIAL TO USE FOR COSMETIC PURPOSES

Some individuals use cosmetics to enhance their features. Other use it to hide blemishes, scars, conditions like Rosacea or wrinkles. Whatever the reason for using cosmetics, it's important to keep skin healthy and clear. One way to achieve this goal is by using essential oils. Using essential oils isn't new or the latest trend. The oils have been used for centuries to help the skin. The following are some of the essential oils used for cosmetic purposes.

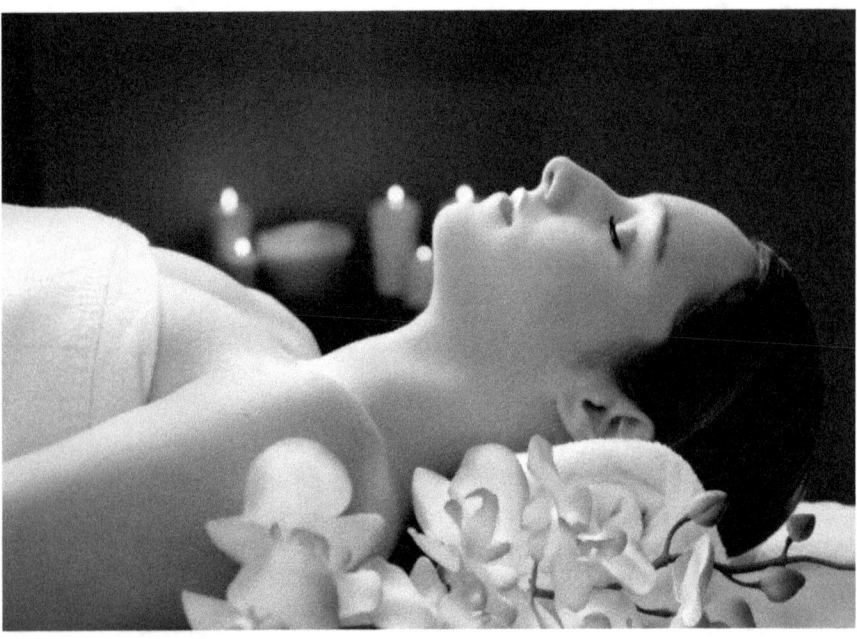

Tea Tree Essential Oil

Tea Tree isn't extracted from a tea plant or any other type of plant. It is extracted from Melaleuca Alternifolia (Tea Tree leaves) and twigs that were steamed and distilled. Besides being a cure-all for fungal infections, dandruff or wounds, it also helps the skin. It helps oily and acne-prone skin. The downside of Tea Tree oil is the smell. It doesn't have a very pleasant smell. So individuals using it may want to combine it with an essential oil that smells good.

Grapefruit Essential Oil

The essential oil in grapefruit is found in its peels. The oils are extracted by compressing the peels to produce a pink, thin oil which has astringent and antibacterial properties. The oil has Limonene and Myrcene as its main components and other things like Sabinene and Geraniol. Like Tea Tree oil, grapefruit oil has a variety of uses. This oil can be used as an antioxidant, diuretic and disinfectant. When used for cosmetic purposes, it removes toxin buildup and rejuvenates lifeless and dull looking skin.

Mandarin Essential Oil

Mandarin essential oil is sometimes referred to as tangerine essential oil because they have the same botanical name of Citrus Reticulata. However, this essential oil is made by using the fresh peel of the mandarin oranges. The process includes extracting the oil via a cold compress. The oil, which contains things like camphene, limonene and nerol, is used in everything from flavoring agent in beverages and food to perfume. When for cosmetic purposes, it helps reduce skin acne. Unlike Tea Tree oil, it smells great.

Helichrysum Essential Oil

Helichrysum is derived from a plant in the sunflower family. Like many other oils Helichrysum is extracted using the steam distilled process. Unlike a many of essential oils, it has a long shelf life. This essential oil is often used for antispasmodic, anticoagulant and antimicrobial purposes. Since Helichrysum essential oil has both anti-inflammatory and antiseptic properties, it's extremely versatile when it comes to cosmetic purposes. For instance, it helps with inflamed, acne and sun-damaged skin.

Lavender Essential Oil

The word "lavender" comes from Lavare which means "to wash." Lavender essential oil comes from the lavender plant. It is also extracted through steam distillation. The health benefits include treating respiratory problems, pain relief and increase blood circulation. Lavender essential oil is most often used to treat acne because it increases the healing and relief. In addition to helping acne, this essential oil soothes inflamed skin and helps dermatitis. It also aids in tissue regeneration.

Elemi Essential Oil

Elemi essential oil comes from the Elemi tree located in tropical forests in countries such as the Philippines. The essential oil has the botanical name of Canarium Luzonicum. To obtain the gauzy oil, it must be weeded out of the gum in the elemi tree. The next process involves extracting it from the gum using steam distillation. Some of the components in the oil include elemol, dipentene, terpineol and limonene.

The non-medical uses for Elemi essential oils include paint, soap and perfume. Health benefits include antiseptic, expectorant, tonic substance, stimulant and analgesic. When used for cosmetic purposes it matures skin and reduces scars.

Vetiver Essential Oil

Vetiver essential oil has the botanical name of Andropogon Muricatus or Vetiveria Zizanoides. Vetiver is a grass which has a pleasant, musky smell. The essential oil is extracted from the Vetiver's root. It has components including vetivenyl vetivenate, beta vetivone, alpha vetivone and benzoic acid. The oil is often used as a room freshener and in perfumes.

The health benefits include soothing inflammation, helping wounds heal and arousing sexual desires. When used for cosmetic purposes, it fades scars and other marks on the skin. In addition, it promotes the growth of new tissues where there were dead tissues. Thus, it creates a uniformed look to skin instead of blotchiness or uneven skin which causes an individual to use more makeup. It's also helpful to women who develop stretch marks during their pregnancy.

Sandalwood Essential Oil

Sandalwood essential oil like other oils is extracted using steam distillation. Makers use wood pieces from Sandalwood trees that are 40 to 80 years old. Older trees are preferred because they have more oil. Health benefits of the essential oil include a diuretic, carminative which helps relief gas and an astringent to strengthen gums and teeth. Sandalwood essential oil is often found in lotions, soaps and creams. It is ideal for soothing skin and fading scars and spots on skin.

This essential oil is extracted from the Camomile plant's flowers. There are two types of Camomile flowers: Roman Camomile and German Camomile. Both have cosmetic benefits when used as essential oils. For instance, they diminish scarring, spots and marks on the face and skin. Another benefit is that they protect the skin from becoming infected when bruised or cut. Camomile essential oil can also be used to fight acne.

It removes toxins and cleans out the eccrine and sebaceous glances that become blocked with sweat. Other health benefits include antibiotic, bactericidal and anti-inflammatory. It helps calm nerves and reduces swelling.

Benefits of Using Essential Oils for Skin

Essential oils are found in many of the daily products used for cosmetic reasons. They assist in preventing breakouts and heal minor skin problems. It's important to be careful when using essential oils. Many are available in highly concentrated form. Thus, they can cause irritation and allergies when too much is used at one time. However, the benefits often outweigh the disadvantages of essential oils.

The Best Sensual Essentials Oil Perfumes

Enhance your sexual appetite with these top ten essential oils. All natural, all earth friendly and all of the best ingredients to heighten the mood and create and romantic setting.

Jasmine

Jasmine is an erotic and floral fragrance that lingers in a subtly yet satisfying way. Jasmine is a popular essence that has been brought throughout history to enhance the sexual arousal in both men and woman. For the female hormones, it is often used for emotional stability during childbirth. Jasmine also relieves the stress that comes with impotence and feeling undesirable.

Ylang Ylang

A gently soft and flowery fragrance accompanies the still enticing bite of this essential oil. Not only does Ylang Ylang enhance the energy between two people, but it has a sweeter scent that plays a calming and relaxing role for nerves as well. Ylang Ylang was used in countries such as Indonesia. Newlyweds would scatter this exotic yellowish flower over the bed for an evening of pure romantic pleasure.

Cardamom

Cardamoms spicy and rich scent brings a heightened new sense of passion. It is an excellent essential oil to include into a passionless relationship. It creates a warming feeling that invigorates the emotional and sensual feelings.

Patchouli

This essential oil has a warm musky undertone that sends any feelings of doubt right out the window.

Coriander

This magnificent spice helps to ease the stress of impotence while stimulating the hormones that are used to create sexual desire.

Neroli

Neroli essential oil is a powerful aphrodisiac that helps decrease stress and anxiety and increase libido in woman.

Cinnamon

Cinnamon with its rush of spicy sensations helps to lift uneasy moods and enhance arousal. Cinnamon has a unique experience that increases blood circulation to stimulate all of the right emotional and physical places.

Agarwood

This essential oil helps to completely relieve stress due to anxiety and depression along with calming nerves that play a role in performance anxiety. This oil prepares the mind and body for a sensual evening.

Lavender

Lavender has always been a great essential oil for calming and easing emotions that often accompany nervousness. Lavender sends a warming sensation to the body that internally rushes blood flow throughout the body evening. It boosts sensitivity in females and a relaxant.

Sandalwood

For the men, Sandalwood will work wonders. It's sweet and woody parts ease tension to allow both parties to open up and become comfortable. It also increases blood flow for stimulation.

Sweet Orange

This is essential oil perfume opens the sense and clears the mind, creating a brighter atmosphere. Sweet orange aroma gives off a sweet citrus scent and can act as an instant relaxant.

Basil

Basil is a popular essential oil that stimulates the mind and allows quick focus. This sweet and herbaceous aroma creates an uplifting atmosphere as while energizes the concentration.

Chocolate Peppermint

A smooth aromatic note of chocolate with the blossoming fume of peppermint sets the evenings into to a whirl. This essential oil is a sweet and cooling refresher that can set a romantic mood the whole night through. Like the traditional uses of peppermint oil, it enhances the sensual sense while relaxing the mind, allowing for extra sensitivity.

Fennel

While fennel has many uses including cellulite and bruise and other ailments, Fennel is incredibly useful for those that do not want a strong scent while trying to increase their sexual moods. This slightly spicy yet sweet aromatic note gives a gentle nudge to your sense, creating a comfortable and sensual experience.

Cypress

Cypress is an essential oil that is not often mentioned but the benefits relating to sensual desire are vibrant. This slightly woodsy and fresh outdoor scent creates an earthy, relaxing and uplifting setting for both men and women.

Geranium

This gentle essential oil provides a very strong sweet and floral note that appeal to the senses. It uplifts the mood and is used to relax and settle nerves while suppresses depressive thoughts and release negatives emotions.

Bergamot

A blend of spicy citrus accompanies antibacterial and non-inflammatory properties that often rise during arousal. Performance anxiety is a common feeling and Bergamot helps reduce the feelings of anxiety and depression.

Rose

A light but floral scent that permeates any room leaving a fresh and comforting scent. Rose essential oil is one the romantic oils that has been used for thousands of years to heighten sensual arousal while balancing the female hormones.

Tangerine

Tangerine stimulates the female and male sensation while reducing stress and relieving anxiety. This sweet yet tangy oil brings a cheery and playful mindset while clearing the mind and body of any negativity that might interfere in sexual activity.

Allspice Berry

This sweet and spicy aroma is warming and comforting. It has a cheering and masculine note that can chisel away even the toughest of moods.

Wild Chamomile

Wild chamomile creates a relaxing atmosphere but stimulates the soothing and nurturing parts as well. It has a clean woody sweet scent that is long lasting.

Clary Sage

Clary sage is a special essential oil that promotes concentration and focus. It centers the mind, sets the mood and relaxes the brain. It is also euphoric and visualizing with a bittersweet aroma.

Frankincense

Frankincense works as a calming and meditative oil that promotes visualization. It centers on focus and mood. It has a floral, spicy and masculine aroma.

Hyssop

This magnificent purifying scent clears the mind and relaxes the muscles. It is a strong sweet and spicy scent with woody undertones. Its refreshing undertone is revitalizing and purifying.

Vetiver

Vetiver oil is sweet and earthy. With a woody undertone, this essential oil helps ease tension, clear moody thoughts and open the mind. It also plays a role in supporting the mindsets natural sensual arousal yet stimulates a grounded feeling as well.

Vanilla

This sweet balsamic essential oil sends a calming very comforting balance for an evening of relaxation and surprise. It is a favorite amongst men and woman because of its very sweet yet satisfying aroma. The feelings of comfort, joy and relaxation are often experienced.

CHAPTER 6- HOW ESSENTIAL OILS CAN BE USED TO ENHANCE WELLBEING

Almond Oil sometimes is combined with other ingredients to enhance its relaxing and soothing properties, nowadays we can find it mixed with lavender in what is known as lavender almond massage oil. The essence of lavender really complements the properties of almond oil.

Lavender essential oil has been used extensively in aromatherapy and it has been known for its relaxation properties. It helps to heal skin, sinuses and lungs. Lavender almond oil cannot only be used in a massage therapy, but it also can be used for your bath time.

After preparing a hot bath, just put a few drops in the water and let the oil vaporize lavender in the air.

If you don't particularly enjoy the smell of almonds, this type of massage oil is a great alternative. It has a particular smell that you won't find anywhere else. After finishing its application through massage you'll enjoy the benefits of having a smoother, softer skin. It is better to opt for organic oils as they are free of impurities in their composition.

If you are worried about remaining sticky after the massage, don't be. This type of oil has the perfect amount of absorption levels, so you'll feel fresh and with a smooth skin afterwards.

Lavender Almond Oil for a Good Night's Sleep?

Many people are starting to use this type of oil as part of a remedy to cure insomnia. It is especially helpful if you suffer from sleeping disorder is linked to anxiety, stress and muscle pain. The directions are the same as the directions to use it during bath time, but make sure bath time is just prior going to bed.

Just add two tablespoons of the lavender almond oil to you bath and enjoy the therapeutic properties of this scent. This same remedy can also be used to heal congestion, aches, sinus pressure and even headaches.

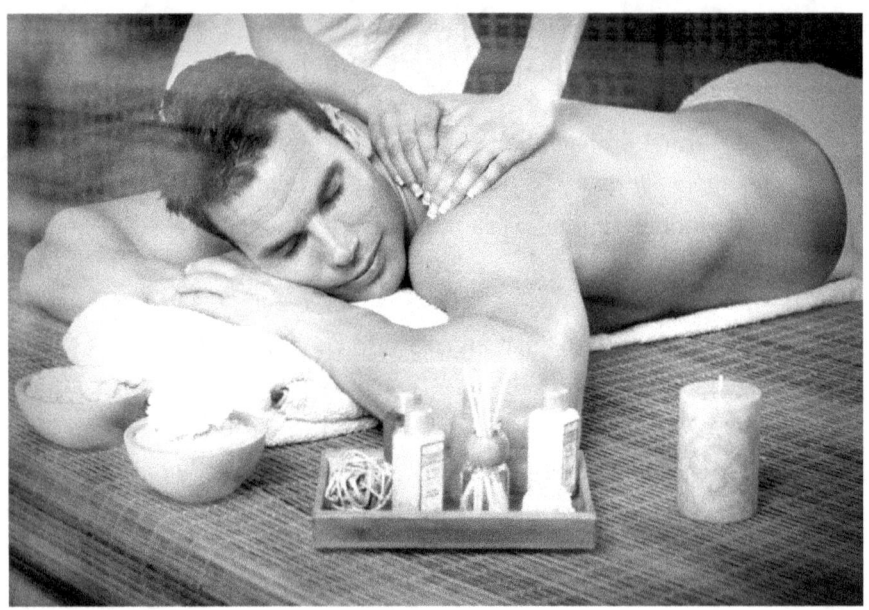

Essential Oil Vanilla for Anxiety

Essential oil vanilla has an awesome scent that is very sweet and soothing, which can ultimately calm one's mind and body. It is considered as one of the most popular aromas due to its comforting and relaxing properties. In fact, this oil is an ingredient of Oriental type perfumes. This oil can also be found in other products, such as candles, air fresheners, body lotions, and bath salts. It offers also numerous benefits to health; it can be a fever reducer, sedative, and anti-anxiety.

The sweet scent of essential oil vanilla carries a calming effect that reduces anxiety. The essential oil of vanilla is extracted from its dried beans. The oil is used in several forms for different purposes. It can be in the form of body lotions, massage oils, lip balms, soap, and other cosmetic products. The aroma of its oil helps in reducing stress and induces sleep. It is also good for skin because it is a powerful antioxidant, which prevents damage of the skin cells due to the toxic actions of pollutants and toxins.

Peppermint Oil for Stomach Aches

Peppermint oil has found to be one of the most popular and versatile oil in existence. It has been known as an effective anti-spasmodic throughout the years. It boosts the digestive system due to the calming effect it brings to other organs of the system. Stomach pains caused by muscle contractions can be relieved with the use of this oil. Many people buy peppermint oil as part of their first aid kits because stomach pains can happen anywhere.

Peppermint essential oil is colorless and has a distinct penetrating scent. It is non-synthetic oil extracted from the peppermint plant and has been used as a tea to calm digestion for many years. Relieving stomach pains is one of the main effects of this essential oil. Its other effects involve mind stimulation to increase focus and mental agility. It is advisable to but peppermint oil as part of your first aid kit.

Frankincense and Myrrh

Myrrh and Frankincense oils are famous around the world not only for its therapeutic uses but are also renowned for its rich history and religious implications. Gold, Myrrh and Frankincense were the gifts given by the three kings to honor baby Jesus. True to its value, Myrrh and Frankincense were considered worthy gifts for they were much more valuable compared to gold! Frankincense is characterized by balsamic-spicy aroma. Myrrh and Frankincense are invaluable to those who take advantage of their therapeutic properties that deals with skin conditions and respiratory ailments.

Myrrh is a brown resinous material collected from dried sap of its trees (Comminphora myrrha). Myrrh is used as a traditionally by many cultures as perfume and medications. It is famous as a remedy for chronic bronchitis and skin ailments such as wounds, acne, and abrasions. Frankincense (Boswellia carteri) is similar with Myrrh in its region of origin. They both are indigenously found in Africa and the Middle-east. Frankincense is incorporated in several fragrances and is also available in its pure form as an essential oil. It has a strong campherous scent that revitalizing and gives a warm feel.

CHAPTER 7- HOW ESSENTIAL OILS CAN BE USED FOR AILMENTS

Cinnamon Essential Oil

Cinnamon is one of the spices mentioned in the Bible; in fact, it was one of the spices God told Moses to take with him from Egypt. And speaking of the ancient Egyptians, they used cinnamon extensively in mummification. Later, cinnamon become so popular in Europe that, at least according to legend, it was the motivating factor behind the discovery of the shipping route around the Cape of Africa.

Characteristics of Cinnamon Essential Oil

Cinnamon leaf oil—the least expensive and more readily available of the two cinnamons in use today— should range from yellow to light brown and have a spicy cinnamon scent with strong overtones of clove. Cinnamon bark oil, on the other hand, should be much darker in color and more viscous texture. This type of cinnamon, which will be far more expensive, will have a strong, true cinnamon scent.

Traditional Uses for Cinnamon Oils

Cinnamon essential oil is still widely used in both the cosmetics and pharmaceutical industries. It's a popular flavoring in oral care products, especially, and performs as a base note in perfumery. Salvatore Battaglia assigns the following therapeutic properties to cinnamon oils:

- Anesthetic
- Antiseptic

- Aphrodisiac
- Anti-Parasitic
- Anti-Microbial
- Stimulant
- Stomachic
- Scientific Studies on Cinnamon Oils

Unlike many essential oils, the various forms of cinnamon essential oil have seen extensive testing for a number of medicinal purposes. Today, for example, we know exactly why cinnamon was so highly prized in mummification—it's a powerful anti-microbial. But cinnamon and the oils made from it have other uses as well.

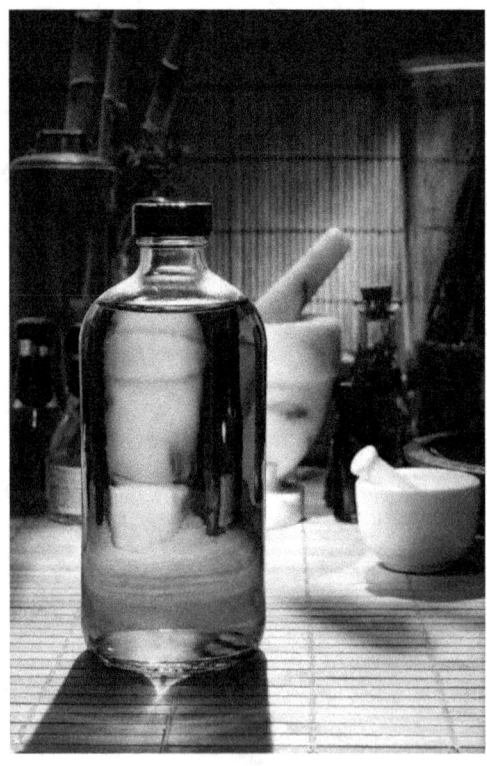

Inflammation

A 2007 study of the major components of cinnamon twig oil led researchers to pronounce that this oil has, in their words, "excellent anti-inflammatory activities and thus have great potential to be used as a source for natural health products".

Anti-Microbial Properties

Cinnamon has long been used as a preservative and today we realize why. Cinnamon oil has been repeatedly shown to have strong anti-microbial properties and can be used to destroy the germs that cause infections like pneumonia, E. coli, lysteria, salmonella and other potentially dangerous diseases.

Repellant Properties

The various cinnamon oils are also proving themselves useful in the fight against some of our most annoying (and in some cases, dangerous) pests. Cinnamon oil has been successfully used to control pests that destroy food crops and pests that pose direct dangers to humans. A 2006 Korean study found that creams made with 5% cinnamon oil provided up to 94% protection against the mosquito that spreads yellow fever among humans.

Safety Issues

Cinnamon oil, especially when it's made from the bark, can be both a sensitizer and a strong dermal irritant. Numerous studies report case after case of allergic-type reactions after topical exposure to various forms of cinnamon oil. This has led some in the aromatherapy community to call for a ban on some cinnamons, especially cinnamon bark oil.

There is also some concern that cinnamon may pose a risk as a lung irritant. A study of workers in a factory where powdered cinnamon was produced found that 87% of them reported some form of discomfort after working around the spice and 22% of them had asthma.

Peppermint

Peppermint has been scientifically proven to have many of the same effects as acetaminophen, one of the most popular ingredients in aspirin everywhere. Unlike a pill, however, you won't ruin your stomach lining with too much of this Christmas favorite. Put a few drops on your tongue to cure a headache; drink it with water to reduce a fever; take a swig straight from the bottle the next time you pull a muscle and need a pain reliever.

Cypress

If you're suffering from muscle spasms and cramps, cypress oil works as an antispasmodic to calm them down. It can also be used to treat the vibrations causing coughs in your respiratory system and the cramping behind all the discomfort in your intestines.

Lemon

Yes, the substance you use to freshen laundry and clean your countertops can also be taken internally! Lemon oil in a nice cold glass of water will help remove toxins and impurities from your system, something sorely needed when your body is under attack. At the same time, it's soothing enough not to upset your digestive system. Some say lemon also has psychological benefits because of its uplifting and instantly recognizable fragrance. It's the kind of scent that perks you up, which is exactly what you want when you're feeling under the weather.

Lavender

Lavender is somewhat of a "cure-all" when it comes to common illnesses and ailments. Not only will it stop sneezes and soothe rashes, but its anti-inflammatory properties can act as a balm to sore throats by relieving some of the pressure of itchy, swollen muscles. It's also great for allergies for the same reason. The next time you sniff a flower only to have your sinuses swell the size of a balloon, take some lavender with a hot cup of tea. You'll feel the results within minutes.

Thieves

This oil blend is made with cloves, cinnamon and rosemary for multiple flu-fighting properties. Originally created by a group of thieves in the 14th century, it was meant to ward off the effects of the Black Plague, but superstition eventually gave way to medicine as doctors realized the mixture really was effective. It just works on coughs, fevers and inflammation, not plagues.

About The Author

Patricia Young has been a licensed aromatherapist since 2001 and she has found it to be the best job that she has had. She loves helping people and finds that through her job as an aromatherapist she can provide that service. Over the years she has discovered that the same essential oils that she uses have so many beneficial properties. This is something that she tries to educate her clients on as they indicate various issues that they have.

As she gained more knowledge on the essential oils that she used in her practice she started to compile a basic guide for persons to read. That soon became a book which could be accessed by persons interested in aromatherapy and the benefits of essential oils.